Asma KEFI
Fatima JAZIRI
Khaoula BEN ABDELGHANI

Infection and Systemic Lupus Erythematosus

Asma KEFI
Fatima JAZIRI
Khaoula BEN ABDELGHANI

Infection and Systemic Lupus Erythematosus

State of the art in an internal medicine department.

ScienciaScripts

Imprint
Any brand names and product names mentioned in this book are subject to trademark, brand or patent protection and are trademarks or registered trademarks of their respective holders. The use of brand names, product names, common names, trade names, product descriptions etc. even without a particular marking in this work is in no way to be construed to mean that such names may be regarded as unrestricted in respect of trademark and brand protection legislation and could thus be used by anyone.

Cover image: www.ingimage.com

This book is a translation from the original published under ISBN 978-620-3-44160-4.

Publisher:
Sciencia Scripts
is a trademark of
Dodo Books Indian Ocean Ltd. and OmniScriptum S.R.L Publishing group
Str. Armeneasca 28/1, office 1, Chisinau-2012, Republic of Moldova, Europe
Printed at: see last page
ISBN: 978-620-5-25532-2

INTRODUCTION

Systemic lupus erythematosus (SLE) is an autoimmune disease of unknown cause that classically affects young women between the ages of 15 and 40. SLE is characterized by a multi-systemic involvement. From remission to relapse, lupus disease acquires its systemic character, resulting in extraordinarily varied clinical pictures due to the multitude of possible associations. From an evolutionary point of view, two types of clinical forms with very different prognoses can be distinguished: benign cutaneous-articular forms and severe forms due to irreversible or uncontrollable damage to a vital organ such as the kidney or the central nervous system (1).

The diagnosis of SLE is based on the presence of 4 criteria from the American College of Rheumatology (ACR) classification criteria adopted in 1982 and revised in 1997, with a sensitivity and specificity of 96% (1).

Infectious complications, although not an integral part of the specific manifestations of lupus disease, deserve to be studied because of their frequency and prognosis. Infections are favored and aggravated by the immunosuppression resulting from the disease itself and from the therapies used.In several series of lupus patients, infections are the leading cause of death, well before renal or neurological causes.It seems that we are witnessing a change in the germs responsible with the development of opportunistic infections (mycoses, viruses, Pneumocystis Carinii) which are often difficult to diagnose post-mortem (1).

Objectives

We conducted a retrospective descriptive study including lupus patients hospitalized between January 2000 and January 2013 with the aim of:

- Determine the prevalence of infectious complications in our patients.

- To study the nature, location and evolution of these infections.

- To compare the demographic, clinical, immunological, therapeutic and evolutionary characteristics of the two groups of patients with and without infection.

METHODS

We conducted a retrospective descriptive and comparative study over a 13-year period between January 2000 and January 2013 in the Internal Medicine A department of Charles Nicolle Hospital. During this period, we included seventy records of lupus patients hospitalized in the department.The diagnosis of SLE was made in all cases when at least four RTA criteria.The positive diagnosis of an infection is based on a combination of clinical, biological and radiological evidence and is confirmed in some cases by the identification of the infectious agent involved (bacteria, virus, fungus or parasite). The information was collected using an information sheet with the following information:

✓ Patient identity

✓ Background

✓ Age of onset of the disease

✓ The different clinical and biological manifestations of lupus disease

✓ Renal biopsy (RBB) was performed in 48 cases. The results

of the anatomopathological study of these biopsies were divided according to the histological classification proposed by the World Health Organization (WHO) (Appendix 1).

✓ Research and titration of anti-nuclear antibodies by indirect immunofluorescence (IFI) on rat liver culture and/or on HEP-2 tumor cells culture.

✓ Identification of native anti-DNA antibodies by indirect immunofluorescence by solid phase assays using Crithidia Luciliae as a support or by enzyme-linked immunosorbent assay (ELISA).

✓ The research of antibodies against soluble antigens was carried out by the ELISA method.

✓ The treatment received by the patients

✓ The different infectious complications presented by each patient with their location, the germ involved, the blood count and the C-reactive protein (CRP) level at the time of infection and the evolution of the infectious episode.

RESULTS

I. DESCRIPTIVE STUDY:

During the study period we included 70 lupus patients hospitalized in our service.

1. EPIDEMIOLOGICAL DATA :

There were 70 patients with SLE, 52 women (74.3%) and 18 men (25.7%) with a sex ratio of 0.34. The mean age at disease onset was 29 years (extremes 7 years and 56 years) (Figure 1).

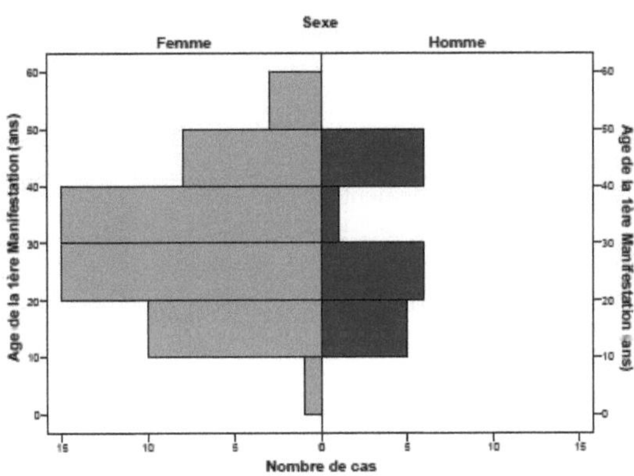

Figure 1: Average age at the start of the LES

2. CLINICAL MANIFESTATIONS:

The prevalences of the different clinical manifestations

occurring at any point in the course are reported in Table 1.

Table 1: Frequency of different clinical manifestations

Clinical manifestationsNumber (%)

Clinical manifestations	Number	(%)
General signs (fever, asthenia, anorexia), weight loss)	37	(52,9%)
Skin involvement	64	(91,4%)
Joint involvement (polyarthralgia +/- arthritis)	63	(90,0%)
Pleural effusion	19	(27,1%)
Heart disease	29	(41,4%)
Kidney damage	60	(85,7%)
Vascular disease	35	(50,0%)
HTA	33	(47,0%)
Venous thrombosis	3	(4,0%)
Arterial thrombosis	3	(4,0%)
Neuro-psychiatric impairment	13	(18,5%)
Hematological disease	53	(75,7%)
Leukopenia	26	(37,1%)
Lymphopenia	40	(57,1%)
Hemolytic anemia	9	(12,8%)
Thrombocytopenia	11	(15,7%)
Digestive disease	14	(20,0%)

We will detail below the serious visceral manifestations:

- **Renal manifestations:**

Renal involvement was manifested in 95% of cases by proteinuria, in 81.6% of cases by hematuria, in 21.6% of cases by nephrotic syndrome and by edema in 58.3% of cases.

Renal failure was found in 63.3% of cases.

PBR was performed in 80% of patients with nephropathy. An involvement of glomerular was found in 100% of cases (Figure2):

- Class I nephropathy in 2.1%.

- Class II nephropathy in 12.5%.

- Class II nephropathy associated with class V in 2.1%.

- Class III nephropathy in 10.4%.

- Class III nephropathy associated with class V in 6.2%.

- Class IV nephropathy in 39.6%.

- Class IV nephropathy associated with class V in 20.8%.

- Class V nephropathy in 6.2%.

Tubulointerstitial disease was associated with glomerular nephropathy in 45.8% of cases. Vascular lesions were associated with glomerular nephropathy in 33.3 % in cases.

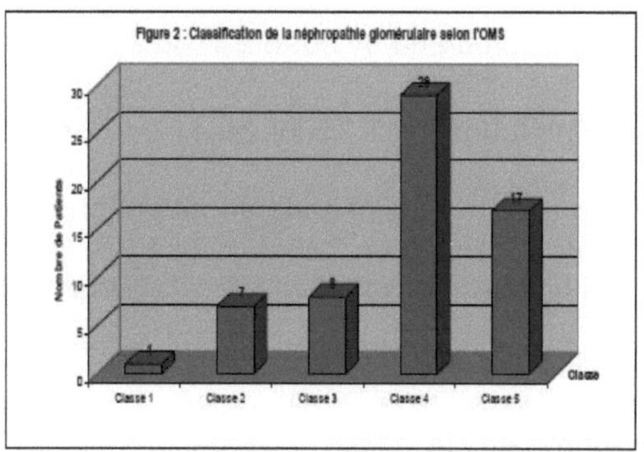

• **Cardiac manifestations:**

Cardiac involvement was observed in 29 patients (41.4% of cases), with pericarditis, myocarditis and endocarditis in 26 cases (37.1%), 3 cases (4.2%) and 4 cases (5.7%) respectively.

• **Neuropsychiatric manifestations:**

These were central neurological manifestations in 10 patients (14.3%), peripheral neurological manifestations in 3 patients (4.3%) and psychiatric manifestations in 8 patients (11.4%).

3. IMMUNOLOGICAL DATA

The search for and determination of NAA was performed in 64 patients (91.4%). They were positive in 96.9% of cases. Anti-DNA and anti-NAA antibodies were positive in 78.6% and 60% of cases respectively.

4. THERAPEUTIC PROFILE

The choice of therapeutic modalities was made according to the different clinical manifestations presented by the patients. Basically, corticosteroid therapy at a dose of 0.5 mg/kg/day was instituted in the treatment of serites and at a dose of 1 mg/kg/day in the presence of autoimmune hemolytic anemia, thrombocytopenia, myocarditis, and renal or neurological impairment.Table 2 represents the frequencies of the different therapeutic modalities.

Table 2: Frequency of different therapeutic modalities

Therapeutic modalities	Number of cases (%)	
Synthetic antimalarials	47	(67,1%)
Systemic Corticosteroid Therapy	63	(90,0%)
Immunosuppressants	36	(51,4%)
Cyclophosphamide	28	(40,0%)
Mycophenolate mofetil	18	(25,7%)
Azathioprine	4	(5,7%)
Plasma exchange	1	(1,4%)
Polyvalent immunoglobulins	4	(5,4%)

II. DESCRIPTIVE STUDY OF INFECTIOUS COMPLICATIONS

Forty-nine of the seventy patients studied developed infectious complications during their follow-up. A total of 96 infectious episodes were diagnosed and the average number of infectious episodes was 2 episodes per patient with extremes ranging from 1 to 6. The mean C-reactive protein level during infectious episodes was 58 mg/L with extremes ranging from 1 mg/L to 326 mg/L.The infection was bacterial in 50% of the cases and viral in 12%, mycotic in 17% of cases and parasitic in 3% of cases (see Figure 3).

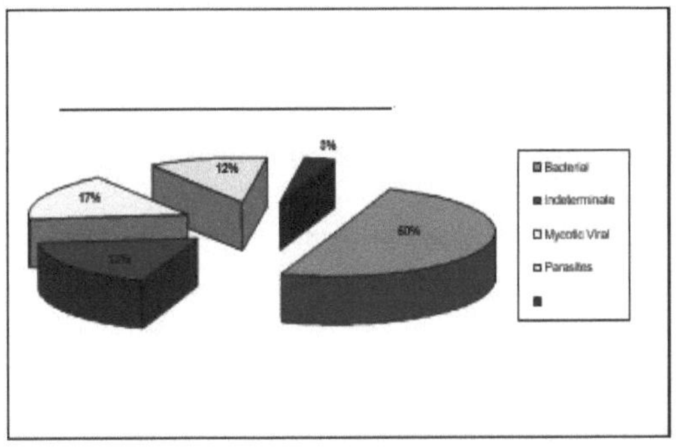

Figure 3: Frequencies of different types of infections

1) Descriptive study of bacterial infections:

Bacteriological examination of urine, sputum, blood cultures and skin samples allowed the isolation of a germ in 29 cases (60%). Gram-negative Bacillus (GNB) and gram-positive Cocci infections were observed in 22 cases (45%) and 7 cases (14%), respectively (see Figure 4). Localizations the most frequently observed bacterial infections were: urinary in 24 cases (50%), sepsis in 8 cases (16%), cutaneous in 8 cases (16%) and bronchopulmonary in 6 cases (12%). There were 3 cases of staphylococcal septicemia, 2 cases of salmonella septicemia, 1 case of enterococcal septicemia, 1 case of streptococcal septicemia and 1 case of enterobacter cloacae septicemia (see figure 5). The evolution of these infections was fatal in 3 patients (6%), following staphylococcal Aureus sepsis in one case, enterococcal sepsis in another case and severe sepsis secondary to febrile gastroenteritis (no isolated germ) in the third case.

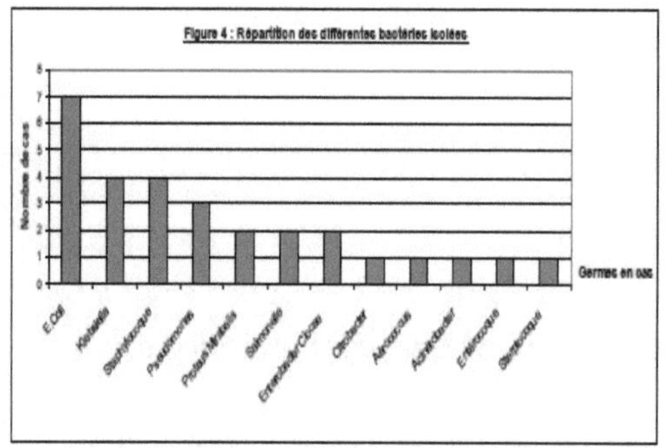

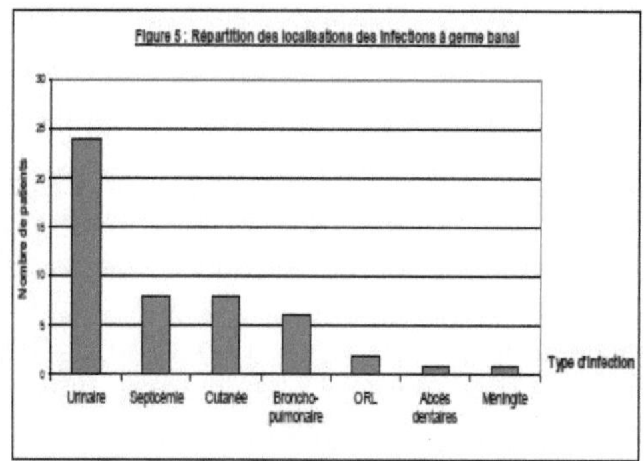

Tuberculosis was diagnosed in 4 patients, bronchopulmonary tuberculosis in 3 cases, including one case of tuberculous miliary and lymph node tuberculosis in the 4th case. The

12

diagnosis was made on the basis of the presence of Koch's bacillus in the sputum of the patients with bronchopulmonary tuberculosis and the presence of granulomatous adenitis with caseous necrosis in the anatomopathological study of the lymph node biopsy in the last case. The evolution was favourable under antitubercular treatment in all cases.

2) **Descriptive study of viral infections:**

Table 3 shows the distribution of the different viruses isolated.

Table 3: Distribution of viruses isolated

Virus	Number of cases
Herpes simplex virus	3 cases
Cytomegalovirus	2 cases
Viral hepatitis B	2 cases
Hepatitis C	2 cases
Epstein Bar virus	1 case
Varicella Zoster virus	1 case
Rubella	1 case

Serodiagnosis allowed us to diagnose viral infections in 8 cases. The localizations of these viruses were hepatic in 5 cases, cutaneous-mucosal in 4 cases and ophthalmic in 1 case. The evolution was favorable under antiviral treatment in all cases.

3) Descriptive study of fungal infections:

It was a candidiasis in 7 cases. The localization of the mycosis was cutaneous-mucosal in 15 cases, esophageal in 1 case and auricular in 1 case. The evolution was favorable in 100% of the cases.

4) Descriptive study of parasitic infections:

Leishmaniasis was diagnosed in 2 patients and was cutaneous in one case and hematopoietic in the other. The evolution was favorable after treatment. Scabies was detected in one patient and progressed well under treatment.

III. Comparative study:

We subdivided our patients into two groups:

• A group of patients who did not develop an infection (group 1).

• A group of patients with infectious complications (group2).

The demographic, clinical, immunologic and therapeutic characteristics of the two groups were compared.

1. Comparison of demographic characteristics of the two groups:

In group 1 there were 21 patients: 16 women and 5 men (sex ratio 0.3), while in group 2 there were 49 patients: 36 women and 13 men (sex ratio 0.36). The difference was not statistically significant ($p=0.8$). Patients in group 2 were younger at the beginning of the disease (mean age 26 years) compared to patients in group 1 (mean age 34 years) with a significant p at 0.01 (figure 6).

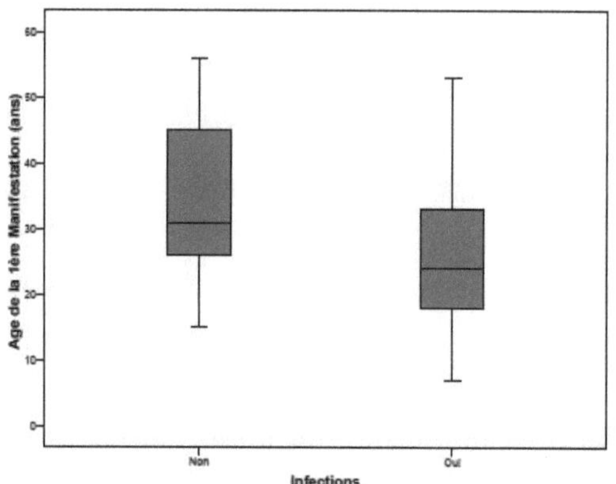

2. Comparison of clinical and immunological characteristics of the two groups:

Table 3 compares the frequencies of key clinical, biological, and immunologic events in the two groups.

Table 3: Comparison of the frequencies of clinical manifestations, biological and immunological characteristics of the 2 groups.

Clinical manifestations	Group 1 n=21	Group 2 n=49	p
General signs	10 (47,6%)	27 (55,1%)	0,565
Skin involvement	18 (85,7%)	46 (93,9%)	0,264
Joint damage	17 (81%)	46 (93,9%)	0,099
Respiratory disease	6 (28,6%)	13 (26,5%)	0,86
Heart disease	10 (47,6%)	19 (38,8%)	0,491
Kidney damage	16 (76,2%)	44 (89,8%)	0,136
Neurological impairment	2 (9,5%)	11 (22,4%)	0,203
Digestive disease	2 (9,5%)	12 (24,5%)	0,151
Hematological disease	16 (76,2%)	37 (75,5%)	0,951
Leukopenia	10 (47,6%)	16 (32,7%)	0,235
Lymphopenia	11 (52,4%)	29 (59,2%)	0,598
Hemolytic anemia	4 (19%)	5 (10,2%)	0,359
Thrombocytopenia	5 (23,8%)	6 (12,2%)	0,126
AAN	18 (90%)	44 (100%)	0,08
Anti-DNA	14 (77,8%)	41 (93,2%)	0,08
Anti-ENA	11 (61,1%)	31 (70,5%)	0,475

ANA: anti-nuclear antibody; anti-DNA: anti-DNA antibody; anti-NAE: anti-soluble nuclear antibody.

3. Comparison of the therapeutic modalities of the two groups:

Table 4 represents the comparison of treatment modalities in the two groups.

Table 4: Comparison of treatment modalities in the 2 groups

Treatment	Group 1	Group 2	p
APS	14 (66,7%)	33 (67,3%)	0,956
Corticosteroids	18 (85.7%)	45 (91.9%)	0,434
Immunosuppressants	9 (42,9%)	27 (55,1%)	0,348
- Cyclophosphamide	7 (33,3%)	21 (42,9%)	0,456
- MMF	3 (14,3%)	15 (30,6%)	0,152
- Azathioprine	0 (0%)	4 (8,2%)	0,178
EP	1 (4,8%)	0 (0%)	0,124
Ig IV	0 (0%)	4 (8.2%)	0,178
Hemodialysi	3 (25%)	14 (33,3%)	0,584

APS: synthetic antimalarials; MMF: Mycophenolate de Mofétil; PE: plasma exchange; IV Ig: intravenous polyvalent immunoglobulin.

4. Evolution in both groups:

In our study, 4 of our patients died; these were in the group of lupus patients who presented infectious complications. Three patients died as a result of sepsis and one patient with advanced renal failure died as a result of acute lung edema.

1. Pathophysiology:

Infectious complications in SLE deserve to be studied because of their frequency and mortality, which have been increasing as therapies such as corticosteroids, immunosuppressive drugs and plasmapheresis have become more and more established (1). In addition to the therapies prescribed during the course of SLE, other endogenous or exogenous factors may promote infections (2-4).

Pathophysiological mechanisms that may explain the increased infectious risks in lupus patients are: Decreased cell-mediated (T-cell) immunity through lymphocytotoxic autoantibodies.

Lymphopenia during relapses.

A genetic determinism: thus the FCγRIIA-R131 genotype involved in the susceptibility to SLE, would predispose to invasive pneumococcal infections by decreasing the clearance of IgG2 opsonized pneumococci.

The presence of functional asplenia. Inherited deficiency in complement factors, in fact the activation of the complement system leads to the formation of the membrane attack complex which is involved in membrane lysis, which is mainly manifested against non-nucleated cells (5). The opsonization of microorganisms or foreign cells by C3b, C3bi (the cleavage product of the C3 fraction of complement by factor I) and C4b allows their attachment to the complement receptors (CR1 and CR3) present on phagocytes and, in a second stage, their phagocytosis. Opsonization/phagocytosis is a mechanism essential notably in the immunity against encapsulated bacteria resistant to phagocytosis.

The C4a, C3a and C5a fragments released during complement activation are called anaphylatoxins because they are capable of causing degranulation of mast cells and basophils, increased capillary permeability and contraction of smooth muscle fibers. In addition, these moieties have a chemotactic role towards cells that possess their specific receptors. C5a is a potent activator of neutrophils and macrophages.

The decrease of the phagocytic power of the polynuclear cells by the decrease of the chemotactic response induced by the complement fraction C5a which is an anaphylatoxin. Indeed, there appears to be an inhibitor of C5a in the serum of lupus patients that specifically blocks the chemotactic function of C5a.

2. Analysis of epidemiological and clinical data:

In our series, the frequency of infectious complications was 70%. This frequency varies between 26 and 78% depending on the series (6), and was estimated at 42% in the Tunisian multicenter study (7). According to several authors, this variability can be explained by numerous factors, including the presence of serious visceral manifestations such as renal damage (2, 6, 8-11) or neuropsychiatric damage (8-12), the activity of lupus disease (8, 10, 11, 13, 14), leukopenia with or without lymphopenia (9, 15), administration of high-dose corticosteroids (dose greater than or equal to 60 mg/day) and/or immunosuppressive treatment, particularly cyclophosphamide, especially when it induces a drop in white blood cells to less than 3,000 elements/mm^3 (2, 11, 14). The higher frequency of infections in our series could be attributed to the higher prevalence of renal involvement in our patients (85.7%), whereas it varied between 40 and 80% in the literature. This is explained by the recruitment of patients, since our department is polyvalent including internal medicine and nephrology. Nevertheless, in our study there was no correlation between the presence of infectious complications and lupus renal disease.

The influence of lupus nephropathy is not unanimous. In the series of Paton et al. which included 102 lupus patients, lupus nephropathy did not influence the incidence of infections (16). Contrary to most authors, we did not find any correlation between neuropsychiatric impairment, hematological impairment, therapeutic modalities and the existence of infectious complications during SLE. In our study, patients in the lupus group with infectious complications were younger at the onset of the disease than patients without infections (mean age 34 years versus 26 years).

This difference could be explained by the presence of complement protein deficiency, in which case SLE manifests itself earlier and is often complicated by recurrent pyogenic infections (17). However, it was not possible to test for complement deficiency in our institution. In recent years, with the development of immunosuppressive treatment, we have seen a modification of the germs responsible for Infectious omplications at course of lupus in favor of opportunistic infections, notably mycotic or viral (1).

3. Analysis of Bacterial Infections:

In accordance with the literature, bacterial infections were the most frequently found in our study (50% of cases). Their frequency varies between 60 and 80% depending on the series (18-20). They are most often recurrent and affect the urinary tract, the lung and the skin in two thirds of cases (2, 21). Other localizations (osteoarticular, central nervous system, endocardium...) are rarer (9). In fact, in our patients, the most frequently observed infectious localizations were urinary (50%), cutaneous (16%) and bronchopulmonary (12%). Sepsis w a s frequently observed in our series (16% of cases). Sepsis was gram-positive cocci in 62% of cases (staphylococcus, streptococcus and enterococcus) and BGN in 38% of cases (salmonella and enterobacter cloacae). Two of the 3 patients who died in the study succumbed to gram-positive cocci sepsis. Indeed, serious infections during SLE are dominated by BGN sepsis but also by staphylococcal sepsis which remains responsible for half of the fatal sepsis in Hellmann's study (1). The incidence of salmonella and pneumococcal sepsis is higher in lupus patients (22). Common bacteria predominate and are responsible for more than 80% of infections in SLE (8,

9).Tuberculosis was detected in 5.7% of our lupus patients, the majority of them being bronchopulmonary tuberculosis with one case of tuberculous miliary. Tuberculosis is reported mainly in endemic countries, with a frequency that varies between 5 and 30% (23). Tuberculosis is more common in patients with SLE than in the general population (24). Indeed, a study by Erdozain et al concluded that the incidence of tuberculosis in lupus patients was six times higher (24). Contrary to our study, tuberculosis infection in SLE is characterized by the frequency of extra-pulmonary localizations (articular, neurological, gastrointestinal or genitourinary) which was estimated at 52.4% in the series by Chih-Lung Hou (25, 26). This frequency is explained by the delay in diagnosis in these immunocompromised patients and the diagnosis is made at the stage of tuberculous miliary and extra pulmonary involvement (27, 28). Tuberculosis is difficult to diagnose, as its presentation is often atypical in the course of SLE and it can be confused with a disease flare (29-31). Pulmonary tuberculosis is also more frequent in lupus patients than in the general population, which is related to the dysfunction of alveolar macrophages and the immunosuppressive treatment of lupus patients (32).

4. Analysis of viral infections:

Some viral infections have been shown to be a trigger for of the disease lupus disease or of a new relapse (33).

The immunosuppression oflupuspatients predisposes themto the occurrence of viral infections, particularly CMV,herpes virus and varicella zoster virus.

The frequency of viral infections was 12% in our series, 12% in the series of Zonana-Nacach et al (6) and 27.7% in the study by Gladman et al (8). In accordance with the literature, herpes virus infections were the most frequent in our study (34). Lupus patients with renal involvement, thrombocytopenia or autoimmune hemolytic anemia or treated with corticosteroids and immunosuppressive drugs are more prone to developing this type of infection (34). Herpes zoster is most often seen in the usual localized form, but disseminated or recurrent forms have been reported in 9 to 15% of cases (34).

Cytomegalovirus (CMV) is a ubiquitous herpes virus in humans. Primary CMV infection is usually asymptomatic and benign in immunocompetent individuals (35). This virus is a major cause of morbidity and mortality, which is well known in transplanted or HIV-positive subjects. In contrast, CMV infection in patients with autoimmune diseases such as SLE and therapeutic immunosuppression is poorly described and less well known. CMV infection in SLE, which is rarer than other herpes virus infections (9), has polymorphous localizations (retinitis (36), colitis (37), pancreatitis (38)). CMV infection can mimic a lupus attack, particularly in the case of digestive localization (39). It was found in two of our patients and was manifested by a prolonged fever. Diagnosis cannot be based on serology alone because anti-CMV IgM is not very specific in lupus (40) due to polyclonal activation of lymphocytes. On the other hand, antigenemia has a sensitivity of 89 to 100% and a specificity of 92 to 96%, allowing early diagnosis (41). Anatomopathological analysis also allows a diagnosis of certainty at the cost of an invasive procedure, except in the case of cutaneous localization(42).

Qualitative PCR is an excellent indication for CSF and aqueous humor; as for quantitative PCR, 50 infected cells correspond to 5.24 log but this technique is expensive and not widely available (41). The diagnosis of CMV disease must therefore be made on the basis of a number of arguments clinical and biological. In our study, the diagnosis of CMV infection was made on the basis of clinical arguments and positive serology. Other means of diagnosis were not available in our institution. The development of biotherapies offers remarkable perspectives in the management of autoimmune diseases but exposes to a greater risk of infections rarely reported until now. Observations of CMV disease have been described with anti-CD20 (43). This infection could therefore become more frequent and should encourage us to rule out the diagnosis in case of suggestive symptoms, particularly in case of hyperthermia or digestive symptoms. Regarding hepatitis B virus infection, which was found in two of our patients, its prevalence seems to be the same in lupus patients regardless of the treatment they are taking and in the general population (44). Most publications have focused on the role of hepatitis B vaccination in the onset of lupus disease or the aggravation of clinical manifestations in these already diagnosed patients (45).

In a prospective study, 28 young Brazilian lupus patients with a low activity score (SLEDAI<4) and receiving low-dose corticosteroid therapy<20mg/day without immunosuppressive treatment were vaccinated against hepatitis B and followed for 7 months. These patients did not develop lupus relapses and did not require an increase in corticosteroid doses or the prescription of immunosuppressive therapy. Also, the efficacy of the vaccine was not impaired in these patients (46).

Hepatitis C virus infection may be associated with connectivities, particularly in the LES (47). There are similarities between the events The clinical features of SLE and the extrahepatic manifestations of hepatitis C virus infection. In our series, hepatitis C virus infection was observed in two patients. Human immunodeficiency virus (HIV) infection has been reported in a few cases. Complete clinical remission of lupus has been reported after HIV infection (48). Emergence of clinical manifestations of HIV infection has been noted in lupus patients after cyclophosphamide therapy (49) and worsening of lupus manifestations has been observed after antiretroviral therapy (50). No cases of HIV infection were observed in our study.

5. Fungal infection analysis:

In our study, candidiasis was the most frequent fungal complication and was mostly mucocutaneous. No case of invasive fungal infection was observed. In the literature, fungal infection is favored by the use of high doses of corticosteroids and immuosuppressive treatment (51). The most common fungal agent found is candida (52).

Localizations are mainly oral, oral-oesophageal and genital (3,13). Invasive fungal infections have been reported in lupus patients and the fungal agents involved were: candida, aspergilus, cryptococcus and pneumocystis (51, 53). Indeed, cases of meningoencephalitis or sepsis due to Cryptococcus neoformans have been observed in lupus patients (53).

Pulmonary pneumocystis is increasingly observed due to the immunosuppression caused by cytotoxic drugs, mainly cyclophosphamide (8, 54).

Pryor et al. reported three cases of pulmonary pneumocystis in a series of 100 lupus patients treated with high-dose corticosteroids combined with cyclophosphamide (54).

Pneumocystis jiroveci (carinii) pulmonary infections have also been described in lupus patients not receiving immunosuppressive therapy (55).

6. Parasitic infection analysis:

In our series, two cases of leishmaniasis and one case of scabies were found. The evolution was favorable in the patients after treatment. The majority of publications have reported cases of visceral leishmaniasis, toxoplasmosis with encephalitic localization and invasive anguillosis (56). These infections pose a diagnostic problem since their initial clinical manifestations may be confused with SLE (57).

The difficulty in diagnosing leishmaniasis is increased by the existence of cross-antigenicity between parasitic antigens and anti-nuclear antibodies (58). A few observations of scabies during SLE have been reported; these were frequently atypical crusted and diffuse forms

(59) and Norwegian scabies, which is favored by long-term corticosteroid therapy course (59).

7. Evolution of infectious complications:

Consistent with the literature (1, 7), infectious complications were the leading cause of mortality in our patients. Surveillance and early detection of infectious outbreaks, vaccination (mainly pneumococcal) and prophylactic use of antibiotics (as for pneumocystis and CD4 lymphopenia) can help to decrease the frequency and severity of infectious complications in SLE (59).

CONCLUSIONS

Infections during SLE are increasingly frequent and constitute one of the main causes of morbidity and mortality.

They are favored by the immunosuppression induced by the disease itself and by the therapies used.

They may mimic a lupus relapse, leading to a delay in diagnosis and treatment. The decisive role of infection in the mortality of patients with SLE makes the treatment of any infectious focus, even latent, indispensable.

Our objective was to determine the frequency and type of infectious complications in lupus patients and to investigate their clinical and evolutionary impact.We conducted a retrospective descriptive and comparative chart review of lupus patients hospitalized in our department between January 2000 and January 2013. The diagnosis of SLE was retained in all cases on the presence of at least four ACR criteria.

The epidemiological, clinical, immunological, therapeutic and evolutionary characteristics of each patient were collected. We were particularly interested in the infectious complications that were observed in the patients included in the study. We noted their types (bacterial, viral, parasitic and fungal), their localization and their evolution. We divided the patients into two groups: group 1 (patients without infection) and group 2 (patients with infection).

We then compared the demographic, clinical, biological, immunological and therapeutic characteristics of the two groups of patients. We thus included 70 patients with SLE, 52 women and 18 men with a sex ratio of 0.34. The mean age at disease onset was

29 years old. Forty-nine lupus patients had an infection at some point in the course of their disease. There were 36 females and 13 males with a mean age of 26 years. The high frequency of infections in our series (70%), could be attributed to the higher prevalence of renal involvement in our patients (85.7%).

A total of 96 infectious episodes were diagnosed and the average number of infectious episodes was 2 per patient. In accordance with the literature, these infectious complications were dominated by bacterial infections found in 50% of cases.

The most common septic locations were urinary (50%), cutaneous (16%) and bronchopulmonary (12%). The most frequently detected bacteria were gram-negative bacilli. Three patients (6%) died as a result of sepsis. Tuberculosis was diagnosed in four cases, including one case of extra-pulmonary tuberculosis. The evolution was favorable in all cases with antituberculosis treatment. Mycotic infections were frequently found in our patients (17%), most often candida infections.

They were of cutaneous-mucosal location in the majority of cases and no patient in the study presented an invasive fungal infection.The viral infections detected in 12% of the cases were mainly herpes virus, which is in agreement with the data in the literature.

The evolution was favorable after specific treatment in all cases. A parasitic infection was found in 3% of the cases, it was visceral leishmaniasis in one case, cutaneous leishmaniasis in another case and scabies in one case.

The evolution was favorable in all cases. Patients in group 2 were younger at the onset of lupus disease than patients in group 1 (26 years versus 34 years with a significant p at 0.01). This could be explained by the complement protein deficiency which predisposes to the occurrence of lupus at a younger age and to recurrent infectious complications.Contrary to most series reported in the literature, we did not find a correlation between the occurrence of infectious complications with severe visceral manifestations and treatment of SLE. Consistent with the literature, infectious complications were the primary cause of death in our series, with 3 of 4 patients dying of sepsis. It is therefore essential to monitor patients in order to detect infectious foci, even latent ones, at an early stage. Some authors advocate vaccination (mainly against pneumococcal disease) and prophylactic use of antibiotics (as for pneumocystis and CD4 lymphopenia) in order to decrease the frequency and severity of infectious complications in SLE.

REFERENCES

1. Meyer O, Kahn MF. Systemic lupus erythematosus. In: Kahn MF, Peltier AP,Meyer O, Piette JC. Les maladies systémiques. Paris: Flammarion Médecine-Sciences, 2001:131-368.

2. Bosch X, Guilabert A, Pallarés L et al. Infections in systemic lupus erythematosus: aprospective and controlled study of 110 patients. Lupus 2006;15:584-9.

3. Kang I, Park SH. Infectious complications in SLE after immunosuppressive therapies.Curr Opin Rheumatol 2003;15:528-34.

4. Neilan BA, Berney SN. Hyposplenism in systemic lupus erythematosus. J Rheumatol1983;10:332-4.

5. Walport MJ. Complement: first of two parts. N Engl J Med 2001;344:1058-66.

6. Zonana-Nacach A, Camargo-Coronel A, Yanez P, Sanchez L, Jimenez- Balderas FJ, Fraga A. Infections in outpatients with systemic lupus erythematosus: a prospective study. Lupus 2001;10:505-10.

7. Louzir B, Othmani S, Ben Abdelhafidh N. Systemic lupus erythematosus in Tunisia. National multicenter study. About 295 cases. Rev Med Interne 2003;24:768-74.

8. Gladman DD, Hussain F, Ibanez D, Urowitz MB. The nature and outcome of infection in systemic lupus erythematosus. Lupus 2002;11:234-9.

9. Jallouli M, Frigui M, Marzouk S, Maaloul I, Kaddour N, Bahloul Z. Infectious complications during systemic lupus erythematosus: a study of 146 patients. Rev Med Interne 2008;29:626-31.

10. Ruiz-Irastorza G, Olivares N, Ruiz-Arruza I, Martinez-Berriotxoa A, Egurbide MV,Aguirre C. Predictors of major infections in systemic lupus erythematosus, Arthritis Res Ther 2009;11:R109.

11. Costa-Reis P, Nativ S, Isgro J et al. Major infections in a cohort of 120 patients with juvenile-onset systemic lupus erythematosus. Clin Immunol 2013;149:442-9.

12. Petri M, Genovese M. Incidence and risk factors for hospitalizations in systemic lupus erythematosus: a prospective study of the Hopkins lupus cohort. J Rheumatol1992;19:1559-65.

13. Noël V, Lortholary O, Casassus P et al. Risk factors and prognostic influence of infection in a single cohort of 87 adults with systemic lupus erythematosus. Ann Rheum Dis

2001;60:1141-4.

14. Jeong SJ, Choi H, Lee HS, et al. Incidence and risk factors of infection in a single cohort of 110 adults with systemic lupus erythematosus. Scand J Infect Dis 2009;41:268-74.

15. Ng WL, Chu CM, Wu AK, Cheng VC, Yuen KY. Lymphopenia at presentation is associated with increased risk of infections in patients with systemic lupus erythematosus. QJM 2006;99:37-47.

16. Paton NI, Cheong IK, Kong NC, Segasothy M. Risk factors for infection in Malaysian patients with lupus erythematosus. QJM 1996;89:531-8.

17. Walport MJ. Complement: Second of two parts. N Engl J Med 2001;344:1140- 4.

18. Khalifa M, Kaabia N, Bahri F, Ben Jazia E, Bouajina E, Omezzine Letaief A. Infections in systemic lupus erythematosus. Med Mal Infect 2007;16 :755-63.

19. Al-Rayes H, Al-Swailem R, Arfin M, Sobki S, Rizvi S, Tariq M. Systemic lupus erythematosus and infections: a retrospective study in Saudis. Lupus 2007;16:755-63.

20. Oh HM, Chng HH, Boey ML, Feng PH. Infections in systemic lupus erythematosus. Singapore Med J 1993;34:4068.

21. Kang I, Park SH. Infectious complications in SLE after

immunosuppressive therapies. Curr Opin Rheumatol

2003;15:528-34.

22. Lim E, Koh WH, Loh SF, Lam MS, Howe HS. Non-

thyphoidal salmonellosis in patients with systemic lupus

erythematosus. A study of fifty patients and a review of the

literature. Lupus 2001;10:87-92.

23. Fessler BJ. Infectious diseases in systemic lupus

erythematosus: risk factors, management and prophylaxis. Best

Pract Res Clin Rheumatol 2002;16:281- 91.

24. Erdozain JG, Ruiz-Irastorza G, Egurbide MV, Martinez-

Berriotxoa A, Aguirre C. High risk of tuberculosis in systemic

lupus erythematosus? Lupus 2006;15:232-5.

25. Hou CL, Tsai YC, Chen LC, Huang JL. Tuberculosis

infection in patients with systemic lupus erythematosus:

pulmonary and extrapulmonary infection compared.Clin

Rheumatol 2008;27:557-63.

26. Feng PH, Tan TH. Tuberculosis in patients with systemic

lupus erythematosus. Ann Rheum Dis 1982;41:11-4.

27. Victorio-Navarra ST, Dy EE, Arroyo CG, Torralba TP.

Tuberculosis among Filipino patients with systemic lupus

erythematosus. Semin Arthritis Rheum 1996;26:628-34.

28. Haanaes OC, Bergmann A. Tuberculosis emerging in patients treated with corticosteroids. Eur J Respir Dis 1983;64:294-7.

29. Darras-Joly C, Wechsler B, Blétry O et al. Tuberculosis disease and systemic diseases. A propos de 16 cas. Rev Med Interne 1998;19:91-7.

30. Millar JW, Horne NW. Tuberculosis in immunosuppressed patients. Lancet 31. 1979;1:1176-8.

32. Kim HY, Im JG, Goo JM, Lee JK, Song JW, Kim SK. Pulmonary tuberculosis in patients with systemic lupus erythematosus. AJR Am J Roentgenol 1999;173:1639-42.

33. Praprotnik S, Sodin-Semrl S, Tomsic M, Shoenfeld Y. The curiously suspicious:infectious disease may ameliorate an ongoing autoimmune destruction in systemic lupus erythematosus patients. J Autoimmun 2008;30:37-41.

34. Kahl LE. Herpes zoster infections in systemic lupus erythematosus: risk factors and outcome. J Rheumatol 1994;21:84-6.

35. Declerck L, Queyrel V, Morell-Dubois S, et al. Cytomegalovirus and systemic lupus erythematosus: a serious

infection of difficult diagnosis. Rev Med Interne 2009;30:789-93.

36. Schlingemann RO, Wertheim-van Dillen P, Kijlstra A, Bos PJ, Meenken C, Feron EJ.Bilateral cytomegalovirus retinitis in a patient with systemic lupus erythematosus. Br JOphthalmol 1996;80:1109-10.

37. Bang S, Park YB, Kang BS, et al. CMV enteritis causing ileal perforation in underlying lupus enteritis. Clin Rheumatol 2004;23:69-72.

38. Ikura Y, Matsuo T, Ogami M, et al. Cytomegalovirus associated pancreatitis in a patient with systemic lupus erythematosus. J Rheumatol 2000;27:2715-7.

39. Ohashi N, Isozaki T, Shirakawa K, Ikegaya N, Yamamoto T, Hishida A.Cytomegalovirus colitis following immunosuppressive therapy for lupus peritonitis and lupus nephritis. Intern Med 2003;42:362-6.

40. Stratta P, Colla L, Santi S et al. IgM antibodies against cytomegalovirus in SLE nephritis: Viral infection or aspecific autoantibody? J Nephrol 2002;15:88-92.

41. Ghigliotti G, Canessa A, Pastorino A, Mazzarello G, De Marchi R, Gambini C. Necrotizing vasculitis induced by cytomegalovirus in a woman with acquired immunodeficiency

syndrome. Ann Dermatol Venereol 1994;121:820-2.

42. Hachfi W, Laurichesse JJ, Chauveheid MP, et al. Acute
cytomegalovirus infection indicative of systemic lupus
erythematosus. Rev Med Interne 2011;32:e6-8.

43. Looney RJ, Srinivasan R, Calabrese LH. The effects of
rituximab on immunocompetency in patients with autoimmune
disease. Arthritis rheum 2008;58:5-14.

44. Abu-Shakra M, El-Sana S, Margalith M, Sikuler E, Neumann
L, Buskila D. Hepatitis B and C viruses serology in patients with
SLE. Lupus 1997;6:543-4.

45. Santoro D, Stella M, Montalto G, Castellino S. Lupus
nephritis after hepatitis B vaccination: an uncommon
complication. Clin Nephrol 2007;67:61-3.

46. Kuruma KA, Borba EF, Lopes MH, De Carvalho JF, Bonfa
E. Safety and efficacy of hepatitis B vaccine in systemic lupus
erythematosus. Lupus 2007;16:350-4.

47. Ahmed MM, Berney SM, Wolf RE, et al. Prevalence of
active hepatitis C virus infection in patients with systemic lupus
erythematosus. Am J Med Sci 2006;331:252-6.

48. Colon M, Martinez DE. Clinical remission of systemic lupus
erythematosus after human immunodeficiency virus infection. P

R Health Sci J 2007;26:79- 81.

49. Hazarika I, Chakravarty BP, Dutta S, Mahanta N. Emergence of manifestations of HIV infection in a case of systemic lupus erythematosus following treatment with IV cyclophosphamide. Clin Rheumatol 2006;25:98- 100.

50. Drake WP, Byrd VM, Olsen NJ. Reactivation of systemic lupus erythematosus after initiation of highly active antiretroviral therapy for acquired immunodeficiency syndrome. J Clin Rheumatol 2003;9:176-80.

51. Fan YC, Li WG, Zheng MH, Gao W, Zhang YY, Song LJ. Invasive fungal infection in patients with systemic lupus erythematosus: Experience from a single institute of Northern China. Gene 2012;506:184-7.

52. Choi SJ, Rho YH, Lee YH, Ji JD, Song GG. Disseminated candidiasis in systemic lupus erythematosus. Clin Exp Rheumatol 2007;25:503.

53. Chen HS, Tsai WP, Leu HS, Ho HH, Liou LB. Invasive fungal infection in systemic lupus erythematosus: an analysis of 15 cases and a literature review. Rheumatology 2007;46:539-44.

54. Pryor BD, Bologna SG, Kahl LE. Risk factors for serious

infection during treatment with cyclophosphamide and high-dose corticosteroids for systemic lupus erythematosus. Arthritis Rheum 1996;39:1475-82.

55. Liam CK, Wang F. Pneumocystis carinii pneumonia in patients with systemic lupus erythematosus. Lupus 1992;1:37985.

56. Alarcon GS. Infections in systemic connective tissue diseases: systemic lupus erythematosus, scleroderma, and polymyositis/dermatomyositis. Infect Dis Clin North Am 2006;20:849-75.

57. Voulgari PV, Pappas GA, Liberopoulos EN, Elisaf M, Skopouli FN, Drosos AA. Visceral leishmaniasis resembling systemic lupus erythematosus. Ann Rheum Dis 2004;63:13489.

58. Sakkas LI, Boulbou M, Kyriabou D, et al. Immunological features of visceral leishmaniasis may mimic systemic lupus erythematosus. Clin Biochem 2008;41:65-8.

59. Ting HC, Wang F. Scabies and systemic lupus erythematosus. Int J Dermatol 1983;22:473-6.

60. Gilliland WR, Tsokos GC. Prophylactic use of antibiotics and immunizations in patients with SLE. Ann Rheum Dis 2002;61:91-2.

APPENDICES

Appendix 1: 1995 WHO Classification of Lupus Nephropathy

✓ Class I: Normal glomerulus by light microscopy and immunofluorescence.

✓ Class II: Pure mesangial glomerulonephritis.

✓ Class III: Segmental and focal glomerulonephritis.

✓ Class IV: Diffuse proliferative glomerulonephritis.

✓ Class V: Extra-membranous glomerulonephritis.

✓ Class VI: Glomerular sclerosis.

TABLE OF CONTENTS